Paleo Diet Plan

Paleo Diet Cookbook Plan for Beginners, Paleo Diet Recipes and Your Own Paleo Diet 7 Day Meal Plan to Help You Lose Weight Quickly and Feel Amazing! (Including Paleo Desserts)

Sara Rider

information is without contract or any type of guarantee assurance.

The trademarks that are used are without any consent, and the publication of the trademark is without permission or backing by the trademark owner. All trademarks and brands within this book are for clarifying purposes only and are the owned by the owners themselves, not affiliated with this document.

TABLE OF CONTENTS

Introduction

I want to thank you and congratulate you for downloading the book, *"Paleo Diet Plan - Paleo Diet Cookbook Plan for Beginners, Paleo Diet Recipes and Your Own Paleo Diet 7 Day Meal Plan to Help You Lose Weight Quickly and Feel Amazing! (Including Paleo Desserts)"*

So you want to get started on the paleo diet because you have heard how good it is and how you can lose a great deal of weight while on this diet. However, do you know what to eat and how to prepare various meals? Adapting a paleo diet will definitely require you to change greatly the foods you eat and how you may prepare various meals. This is however not to scare you but rather to inform you of the changes you would need to make.

This book has provided you with over 35 Paleo recipes that you can make today. You will also have access to a 7-day meal plan to give you an idea of how you can adapt a paleo diet in your day to day life. The bonus that this book offers you is that you have two plans which you could use! All you need to do is to understand which plan works best for you when you test it! You could then use the different recipes that have been given in the book to create your own plans. I assure you that this book is all you need to get started on your paleo diet.

Thanks again for downloading this book, I hope you enjoy it!

Chapter 1:
What is the Paleo Diet?

Paleo and the Paleo Diet

The word paleo is a derivative of the word 'Paleolithic'. What we call this is not half as important as the power involved with this idea. In recent times, people have begun to understand the importance of having a diet similar to the ones our ancestors had. The term paleo has become popular ever since. It is a known fact that our ancestors suffered from lesser chronic diseases than we do in the modern world. They essentially led healthier lives. This is accountable mainly to the fact that they only consumed "real food". What we mean by real food is the food that provides our body with the essential nutrients and strength. It is impossible for us to eliminate all the pollution around us and create an environment like theirs. We must adapt to this environment around us and start following a paleo diet.

When we say that we need to follow a paleo diet we do not mean that we must replicate the diet the cavemen followed exactly. We need to consume food that will provide us with all the required nutrients so that we can live a healthy life. In essence, we need to implement a balanced diet in our lives. There are no rules that state that if you start following a paleo diet you must give up on dairy products or start consuming low carbs. Keep the following two points in mind when you are following a paleo diet.

1. Consume only whole and unprocessed food. This type of food is extremely rich in nutrients and also provides our bodies with a lot of energy. In addition to this, they also help in strengthening your immune system. This

category of food includes meat, eggs, fruits, nuts, seafood and vegetables. Look to purchase the non-processed varieties. This will eliminate the possibility of chemicals entering your body through food.

2. Keep away from foods that can mess up our metabolic processes. Avoid the consumption of large amounts of gluten. Sugar is another item to stay away from. Also avoid artificial foods.

It is believed by many nutritionists, physicians and other researchers that our ancestor's diets were a lot more nutritious and hence had a greater benefit to humans. It has also been found that people who have implemented paleo-diets have greater health and immunity. They have greater fitness and energy levels. Apparently, people who follow such approaches have lesser susceptibility to a various number of diseases as compared to those who consume normal diets.

The Myth behind the diet

When it comes to following the paleo diet, all evidence points in favor of it. Some people however get a little worried when it comes to longevity – it is believed that cavemen rarely lived for more than 30 years. What must also be remembered is that cavemen did not live in the same conditions that we live in now.

They had to look around for shelter whereas we have homes we can go back to every day. They had to live in the wild and were constantly surrounded by carnivores. Safety was a major issue for them. Considering that the adults had to protect their younger ones from these dangers, it isn't a surprise that they rarely lived beyond 30. Also, we have made massive advancements in the field of medicine. We have medicines for even tiny illnesses. They had none of that to cure them. Infant mortality rate was higher too those days. Of course, a few cavemen lived way beyond the age of 30. The average age that they lived up to however, is believed to be around 30 years.

Three Simple and Stringent Rules to Follow

With most diets, people find it very difficult to the diet they have decided for themselves- be it a weight loss diet or weight gain diet. This is not the case when it comes to a paleo diet though. It is mandatory that you must reduce the amount of junk food you intake but it isn't very stringent in that it doesn't necessitate a low carb or low fat diet. You can create a Paleo diet using any of the natural food around you. There are tons of delicious foods that you can include in your Paleo diet. There are many recipes that you can follow in order to make good food so that your Paleo diet is easier to stick to. In order to stick to your Paleo diet, you need to follow three very simple rules that have been given below.

Always stick to the plan!

As with any other diet, there might be times when you stray from your paleo diet. There will obviously be times where you just want to eat junk food or consume sugary foods. You can do it once in a while but get back to your paleo diet immediately. Try your best to avoid junk and processed food.

Follow the motto of KISS (Keep it simple silly)

Make sure that your plan is simple and extremely easy to follow. Do not make it too strict because you will end up dropping it. Ensure that the food you have included in your diet is easy to prepare because if you are a very busy person you will not have time to prepare complicated meals and you will end up giving up the Paleo diet.

Make sure that the food you consume is delicious!

As mentioned earlier, the food that is included in your paleo diet need not be food that is not tasty. This will only make it harder for you to stick to your diet. People fear that they will have to stop eating all of their favorite foods if they take up a paleo diet. This is not true. All you need to do is consume less oily food and also do not consume too much of fatty food.

Things to keep in mind

By now, you have probably understood the meaning of the words "paleo diet" and are also aware of what its implications are. Listed below are three things you need to keep in mind once you have started on your diet.

This is not only for weight loss

Quite a few people have unwanted fat in their body because they have indulged in a variety of junk food throughout their lives. You must remember that a paleo diet is not primarily a weight loss diet, i.e. taking up a paleo diet doesn't mean that you will get rid of the unwanted fat. You will, however, become healthier and will have a better body composition. Do not rely on this diet to lose weight.

Test the plan for a week

It is obviously difficult to stick to your paleo diet initially because you are accustomed to the diet that you have been following for so long. People will miss the food that they have been consuming and will begin craving for junk food. You must fight this urge and stick to your diet. After around a week or 10 days it will become easy to stick to your diet.

Make sure you eat the right way!

At first glance, you might feel that this type of diet is highly restrictive. However, if you compare this diet to other types of diets you will see that it is a lot more flexible. It allows you to eat a variety of foods that provide you with nourishment and energy. You can include fats in your diet as long as they are of the healthy kind. It is easier to stick to a paleo diet than say, a weight loss diet.

Chapter 2:
Understanding the Science Behind the Diet

Although it has been mentioned that the Paleo diet is flexible, there are quite a few foods that you will be asked to avoid. You may question why you need to stop eating foods that are so tasty and have also been consuming for so long. This chapter gives reasons as to why you need to quit the foods that you have been consuming.

Gluten

The reasons for not consuming large amounts of gluten need not be stated because it is rather obvious. What exactly is gluten? Gluten is a mixture of proteins that we find in quite a few of the foods we eat. Most commonly, it is found in wheat, barley and rye. It is found in almost all the baking goods (because they somehow incorporate wheat). It is used in the making of dough because it provides the dough with elasticity and makes it rise and retain its shape. Therefore, most bakery products have gluten in them.

Gluten has become a very common term used by people off late. Awareness about the disadvantages of gluten has risen. People have started learning that the consumption of large amounts of gluten will end up causing a number of digestive problems. Some of the problems it may cause are acid reflux, constipation, bloating and diarrhea. The immune system and endocrine system need to get involved in order to cure these illnesses. Hormonal imbalances may occur and it may also lead to inflammations in certain areas or a fever. This may also lead to the onset of joint pains. Worst case scenario, it may even affect the menstrual cycle in women.

Phytic Acid

Phytic acid is a saturated cyclic acid and is the principal form of storage of the element phosphorous in plants. It is found mainly in grains and nuts. Our body lacks an enzyme called phytase which is essential to digest phytic acid. The molecules of phytic acid stick to various minerals such as magnesium, iron, calcium and zinc. It sticks to them anywhere; even if the minerals are present in the intestine. The effect of this is you're your body is unable to assimilate these minerals and these minerals are just excreted out. This causes a deficiency of these minerals in your body which leads to deficiency diseases. You may be consuming foods that are rich in these minerals but due to the consumption of grains, the phytic acid content in your body increases. Due to this your body lacks in calcium or magnesium content. It is believed that this acid is the primary factor that causes people to be anemic.

Nuts and Seeds

It was mentioned earlier in the book that a Paleo diet requires you to eat more nuts and seeds. Isn't this surprising then? Why does this book now say that you must avoid consuming too many of them? In all honesty, nuts and seeds are quite harmful to your body. They contain a large number of tiny molecules of lectins and phytic acid.

However, there is a way to consume these nuts and seeds without them having many effects on you. The method requires you to soak the nuts and seeds that you want to eat. You need to soak them until they sprout. The soaking helps in eliminating all the lectins and phytic acid present in the nuts and seeds. Hence, they become less harmful to the human body. There are certain procedures that you must follow while soaking the nuts and seeds. You can look these up online.

Try as hard as you can to avoid consuming nuts and seeds (even if they are soaked). Never exceed more than an ounce per day. Since a paleo diet is meant to somewhat resemble the diets of our ancestors, think about it this way- did our ancestors have access to all nuts and seeds like we have now? Probably not; so you need to consume as less of these as possible as well. Also consume fewer amounts of products that are derivatives of nuts such as peanut butter and almond cookies. They contain a large amount of nuts and can harm your body.

Although a paleo diet asks you to include nuts and seeds in your diet, it gives more emphasis to other foods such as fruits, vegetables, sea food and meats. So you should consume more amounts of these foods as compared to nuts and seeds. Nuts and seeds have a large amount of essential nutrients but in large quantities, they can have adverse effects on your body so it is advisable to consume them only in small amounts.

Grains

The inclusion of grains in this list must be very surprising because it is such a common food. Tons of people around the world have been consuming grains for a very long time. Then why are we asking you to stop consuming them? Here's why:

The main constituent of grains more often than not happens to be wheat, wheat flour or white flour. Some examples of grains are rice, barley, rye, corn, millets, oats and buckwheat. A number of foods that we consume often include grains- bread, cereal, cookies, pasta, beer and other alcohols. Quite a number of foods like soup include grains in them for thickening. Most of the prepackaged foods include grains in them as well. These are some of the most common foods in almost everyone's diets. Here is why you need to avoid including them in your diets.

The main nutrient in grains is carbohydrates and they contain a large amount of carbs. It is difficult for the digestive system to break down carbohydrates. When they are not broken down entirely, they occupy a large amount of space for storage. Due to this, you do not feel full and you end up getting hungry in between meals. You begin snacking and this only adds to the unwanted fat in your body. This will eventually lead to obesity.

Legumes

When compared to grains, legumes or beans are not that harmful. However, these also contain considerable amounts of gluten and other harmful substances and should not be consumed in large amounts. They can be consumed if they are cooked properly for a long time. It is advisable to only consume legumes that have sprouted well and fermented. These processes help in removing many of the lectins and phytic acids.

One of the most well-known legumes is soy. This is not processed appropriately in many countries around the world. Due to this, many of the toxins are not eliminated and consuming soy becomes harmful. Soy has a high content of plant based estrogen. This is a hormone that can be harmful to both men and women. In recent times, discoveries have been made to artificially manufacture soy through genetic modifications. However, many studies have been conducted which prove that these artificially generated legumes are very harmful to the body's immune system. They also increase the amount of gas in the body.

Some Lectins

Lectins are everywhere. They are present in each and every food that we consume. They are present inside us as and every other living being as well. They are proteins that help in protecting living beings against diseases. They also aid the animals and plants in protecting them against human beings. For instance, there is a lectin present in wheat known as wheat germ agglutinin or WGA. This is found mostly in the seeds, grains, nuts and beans. These lectins have a very sticky surface. When consumed, they go right down to the small intestine and latch onto the inner lining. They trick the host organism into thinking that they are beneficial to the body. Due to this they are carried down to the border of the tract by the intestine. At this point your body realizes that these are not actually essential and starts producing antibodies to destroy them. When a body creates an antibody, it retains the memory on how to generate the antibody so that it can produce it immediately the next time there is an attack.

Lectins start molding themselves so that they start resembling the organs in your body. Your body has already created antibodies against these lectins. So, it starts to produce these antibodies again and they start attacking the organ that the lectin resembles. This leads to a number of autoimmune diseases such as rheumatoid arthritis and celiac.

Vegetable Oils

You might be wondering what exactly vegetable oils are. It is a common misconception that these oils are extracted from vegetables. The truth, however, is that they are neither made out of nor extracted from vegetables. These oils are extracted from seeds. It is not an easy job to extract them.

These vegetable oils contain a large number of fats. These fats, when oxidized, tend to cause a large amount of inflammation in various parts of the body. The fats can also lead to a number of heart illnesses. They can also be the root cause for chronic inflammations in the body. Not many years ago, vegetable oils were widely believed to be very good for health. However, in recent times, it has been discovered that these oils have a large number of omega 6 fats which have adverse effects on a person.

Try to consume oils other than vegetable oils. There are many oils out there that do not contain harmful amounts of omega 6 fats and hence do not have too harmful an effect on you. Two of the most common substitutes for vegetable oil are coconut oil and olive oil. These are probably already used a lot at your home for cooking and other domestic purposes.

Refined Sugar

Sugar itself is a sweet substance. Refined sugar is further sweeter. This substance is a form of a simple carbohydrate. They are generally made out of maple syrup, sugar cane, honey, beets and corn. When these are processed and chemically altered, they form refined sugars. Some of the more common refined sugars are refined honey, refined maple syrup and white sugar.

There are tons of products that we consume quite often that contain corn syrup and white sugar. Most people are aware of this fact. Right from almost every soft drink like cola to candy bars to biscuits; everything has some amounts of either corn syrup or white sugar. These sugars would never have become an issue had we not started consuming such great amounts of these products. Since we consume so much of these sugars, their harmful effects have come to light and they have now become a problem.

As you consume such large amounts of the sweet products, what you are doing is increasing the sugar level in your blood. This has adverse effects on your body. When blood contains excess sugar it becomes toxic. Now, to balance this out, your body releases insulin- a hormone which converts glucose to glycogen (storage form of glucose). This insulin goes to the cells in your body. It stimulates them to convert the glucose present in the surrounding blood into glycogen. Essentially, insulin helps in regulating the blood sugar levels. However, since so much glucose has been stored your body never gets around to using all of it. It is rarely converted to energy and is just stored as glycogen. The glycogen now gets converted to fat and starts accumulating in different regions of your body as unwanted fat. Also, since sugar is just a carbohydrate you end up feeling hungry quite soon after consuming these products. This will lead to you over eating and will also contribute to your body fat. You also feel tired after consuming these products. So you have an energy drink or some caffeine product in order to get energized. These products release adrenaline and cortisol in your body.

This released cortisol is a hormone and it starts to stimulate the glucose that has been stored in your cells. The glucose is now released into your blood stream in order to give you energy. The adrenaline gives you a feeling of exhilaration (fight or flight). It basically makes you feel like you are faced by a near death experience. If you continue to consume large amounts of sugar you will face a number of issues. Two of the more serious issues have been elaborated on below:

1. Cells in your body will cease to respond to the insulin hormone. Most of the insulin that your body will release from that point forward will simply be absorbed by the cells and glucose will not get converted. So, the blood sugar level shoots up and this leads to diabetes. This is the reason why diabetic people need to give themselves insulin shots.

2. This second consequence of large sugar consumption is quite serious. It is a chronic secretion of the cortisol hormone. This hormone can basically control your immune system and endocrine system (which in turn regulate other systems such as the reproductive system). It is to these systems what a captain is to a sports team. It could end up shutting your immune system down entirely.

It is very simple to avoid the above issues- just avoid consuming foods that can increase your blood sugar level in large quantities. It is definitely easier said than done. Implementing a paleo diet will help you in this endeavor. You cannot entirely give up on sugar. You need some amount of sugar in your daily diet. Just do not let the consumption levels borderline on dangerous and fatal. If you continue to do this, you will be harming your body in numerous ways. In addition to diabetes, excess sugar will also make you over weight. You will also become lethargic. You will feel tired and lazy throughout the day even though you may not have done too much work. You may also go into depression. It will also ruin your teeth and cause other oral issues.

Chapter 3:
Changes to Expect While on the Diet

A paleo diet is versatile in nature. It can help in reducing weight and also helps in balancing the metabolism rates of the body. It provides the body with an all-round transformation. It increases the amount of energy in your body and makes you feel fitter. We have listed a few of the changes that you may experience when you take up a paleo diet. These changes have been scientifically proven. Make sure that you keep a track of these changes which will help motivate you in the future when you find yourself craving for food that you should not eat on this diet.

Muscle gain

Since this diet is rich in proteins you will be able to gain good muscle while you are following a paleo diet. So, if you are someone who goes to the gym regularly, you will find that your muscles grow better and are also toned better when you follow a paleo diet. This diet provides your body with all the necessary nutrients. It will help you stay fit and stay healthy. In addition to strengthening the muscle fibers, this diet also helps in increasing the amount of good fat that surrounds your muscles.

Effortless Weight loss

As mentioned earlier, a paleo diet includes whole foods, i.e. heavy and filling foods. Once you embark on a paleo diet you will notice that you do not feel very hungry in between meals as you normally do. You will start eating lesser junk food and in the process you drop some weight.

Better Libido

Since this diet helps you to drop unwanted weight without much effort you begin to feel much better both mentally and physically. Your self-confidence also increases. Your hormones attain a balance. You also find yourself feeling a lot more calm and composed.

Increased fertility

Another common component of paleo diets is leafy green vegetables. These vegetables increase the amount of leptin in your body which is a substance that has a direct impact on your fertility. Grains and other foods rich in carbs decrease the amount of leptin in your body and it is advisable to avoid them. These foods will have consequences later on in life.

Clear Skin

Another advantage of a paleo diet is that it helps in attaining clear skin. Most paleo diets do not include food that have a lot of sugar. The nutrients such as vitamins and other minerals present in the meat that you have in your diet are perfect for your skin. It helps in clearing up your skin and it also prevents acne and pimples.

Better digestion

A paleo diet generally includes foods that are rich in proteins and carbs. Amino acids that are present in the proteins help in slowing down the metabolism of the carbs and provide time to the food present in the alimentary canal to pass through freely. These diets also include high amounts of fiber and this helps in preventing constipation.

Good Sleep

The sea food and meat included in the diet are good sources of the hormones melatonin and serotonin. These two hormones regulate your sleep cycle. Hence, it is important to have good amounts of this hormone in your diet in order to have a good sleep. In addition to this, serotonin gives a feeling of elevation which leaves the person happy and provides a feeling of being "at peace".

Chapter 4:
What to Eat and What to Avoid

Before we get started, it is important to look at what to eat and what you need to avoid while on the Paleo diet. While some people may think that your options are very limited on the paleo diet, this is actually not the case. What I love most about the paleo diet is that it will make you get out of your comfort zone and make you explore other amazing foods that you have never thought to try because you were too busy eating grains mostly. Here are some foods that you can eat:

- Grass produced meats

- Fish and other sea food

- Eggs

- Healthy oils like avocado, macadamia, walnut, coconut and olives

- Nuts and seeds

- Fresh fruits and vegetables

Foods to Avoid

- Legumes

- Refined sugars

- Refined vegetable oils

- Any type of dairy

- Salt

- Cereal grains

- All processed foods

- Alcohol

With that in mind, let us look at some paleo recipes.

Chapter 5:
Paleo Breakfast Recipes

Zucchini Pancakes

Servings: 2

Ingredients

- ½ zucchini, shredded

- ½ cup almond flour

- 1 egg

- ½ tsp. dried parsley

- ½ tsp. dried basil

- Salt and Pepper to taste

- 1 tbsp. Butter

Directions

Take a small mixing bowl and add the shredded zucchini to it along with the almond flour and the basil. Add the parsley and salt and pepper to the bowl and mix the ingredients well together. Add the egg to the bowl and mix the ingredients well together. Make a few patties with the dough you have. Take a medium sized pan and add the butter to the pan. Once the butter has melted, add the patties to the pan and cook them well on both sides. Once they have turned brown, serve them hot!

Chicken Salad

Servings: 2

Ingredients

- ½ lb. of chicken

- ¼ cup dried cranberries

- ½ cup low fat mayonnaise

- 1 tsp. lemon juice

- Salt and Ground pepper to taste

Directions

Take a large bowl and add the chicken to the bowl and fill the bowl with water while ensuring that the chicken has been covered well. Once the chicken has been boiled well, cut it into small pieces and add it to a small mixing bowl. Add the cranberries to the bowl and mix it well with the chicken. In a smaller bowl, mix the ground pepper, salt, mayonnaise and the lemon juice. Ensure that the mixture has blended well. Now add this mixture to the chicken and the cranberries. Make sure that the ingredients have been coated well with the dressing. Leave it in the refrigerator and serve it cold.

Scrambled Eggs

Servings: 4

Ingredients

- 6 eggs

- 4 tbsp. low fat coconut milk

- 2 tsp. Coconut oil

- Salt and Pepper to taste

Directions

Crack the eggs in a large mixing bowl while ensuring that pieces of the shell are not in the bowl. Whisk them or beat them well while keeping in mind that there should not be too many bubbles. Add the pepper and the salt to the bowl and mix it well. Now add the coconut milk to the bowl and beat the eggs once more while ensuring that there are no bubbles formed. Place a non – stick pan on a medium flame and add the coconut oil to the pan. Once the oil has heated, add the coconut mixture to the pan and let it cook for a minute before you start stirring the mixture. You will need to continue to stir in the direction you began with. Once the eggs have been cooked well, you will need to let the mixture cool and add the salt and pepper to the mixture.

Eggs Baked in Avocado

Servings: 2

Ingredients

- 1/8 teaspoon of pepper

- 1 tablespoon of chopped chives

- 4 fresh eggs

- 2 ripe avocados

Directions

Preheat the oven to 425 degrees F. Meanwhile slice both avocados in halves and take out the seed in the middle. Scoop out a bit of flesh from the center of the avocado so that the egg fits in perfectly. Place the pitted avocados in a fitting bowl and crack the eggs in the pit of the avocados. Try your best to first let the yolk pour out so that the whites fill in the left space. When the avocados are filled to the brim, place them in the preheated oven and let it bake for 15-20 minutes. However, the overall time will depend on the size of your avocado and eggs, so you should be checking them frequently. When they are through, remove from oven, and garnish as you may wish

Kale and Red Pepper Frittatas

Servings: 2

Ingredients

- ½ cup onion (chopped)

- 3 slices bacon (chopped)

- 1 tbsp. coconut oil

- ½ cup red pepper (chopped)

- 2 cups kale (chopped, rinsed and de – stemmed)

- 4 eggs

- ½ cup coconut milk

- Salt and pepper to taste

Directions

Before you begin the process, you will need to preheat the oven to 250 degrees Fahrenheit. While the oven is heating, take a small mixing bowl and add crack the eggs carefully in the bowl. Beat the eggs well together and ensure that the mixture is a light yellow with no bubbles. Now, add the coconut milk to the mixture while whisking the two together. Next, add the salt and pepper to the mixture and mix it well. Leave this mixture aside and place a medium sized pan on a low flame. Add the coconut oil to the pan and when the oil has heated well enough, add the onions and sauté them well. Add the red peppers and sauté them as well. Once the red peppers and the onions have been cooked, you will need to add the Kale and cook it till the leaves have begun to wilt. Add the mixture of the eggs to the pan and add the bacon strips to the pan. Once the bottom of the mixture has been set, you can remove the frittata off the gas and cook it in the oven for twenty minutes. Once it has cooled down, make slices and serve it warm.

Spicy Sausage with Broccoflower

Servings: 2-4

Ingredients

- 1 broccoflower floret (or cauliflower can be substituted)

- 1 pound hot Italian sausage

- ½ cup of chopped parsley (fresh)

- 1 cup of red bell pepper (diced)

Directions

Heat a large pan over medium heat. Remove all the casing from the Italian sausage and put the sausages in the pan. As you cook, break the sausages into pieces using a spatula and let it cook until it's brown. Chop the broccoflower into very small florets and put them in an 8x8 glass dish. Cover it with some plastic wrapping on top and place the dish in a microwave. Set the microwave on high and cook it for a few minutes making sure you don't overcook it. You could also steam the broccoflower for a few minutes instead of cooking it. Now add the broccoflower to the sausages in the pan and cook for 5-10 minutes while stirring. Put out the heat and set the meal on a plate. Add the red pepper and parsley to taste and serve while warm and enjoy.

Sweet Potato Hash

Servings: 8

Ingredients

- 4 onions (sliced)

- 8 tbsp. olive oil (keep the oil divided into two small cups or bowls)

- 2 tbsp. ghee

- 6 Italian sausages (diced)

- 6 sweet potatoes

- 4 twigs of rosemary

- 8 eggs

- Salt and pepper to taste

Directions

You will first need to preheat the oven to 450 degrees Fahrenheit. Place a medium sized skillet over medium flame and add one cup of the olive oil to the skillet. Once the skillet has warmed, add the onions and sauté them till they are translucent. Add the salt to the skillet and turn the flame low. Let the onions turn a light brown and start peeling the potatoes. Cut the potatoes into little cubes and add these potatoes to the mixing bowl. Add the rosemary and the other cup of the olive oil to the mixing bowl and mix the ingredients well to ensure that the potato is marinated well. In another skillet, start cooking the Italian sausages. Cook them till they turn a light or a dark brown. In another mixing bowl, add the

Italian sausages and the onions together. Add salt and pepper to the mixture and balance the taste. Line a baking tray with a parchment sheet and add the potato to the tray and roast it in the oven till the potatoes are soft and brown. Add onions and the Italian sausages to the skillet followed by the potato. Create a few holes in the skillet and add crack the eggs in the wells. Add a little salt and pepper to the eggs and let them cook well together. Serve it hot!

Paleo French toast

Servings: 6-8

Ingredients

- 1 pinch of sea salt

- 1 loaf of Paleo banana bread

- ¼ cup of almond or coconut milk (optional)

- 4 eggs

- 1 teaspoon of cinnamon

- Any healthy oil of your choice

Directions

Make any Paleo banana bread whenever (below is a recipe you can use). This can be done the night before and refrigerated to be used in the morning or prepared in the morning. Start by slicing the already made banana bread to slices (1/2 inch slices). Place your skillet over medium heat and let it heat up. As it heats, add the sea salt, coconut/ almond milk, eggs and cinnamon in a mixing bowl and beat until the mixture is well scrambled. When the skillet is fully preheated, smear your desired oil all around. Deep the slices one by one in the egg mixture and make sure that every inch of the bread is covered with the mixture. Place the coated bread in the skillet and let it cook on each side for 3-4 minutes. When it is perfectly cooked, remove it from the skillet and set it on a plate. Garnish it with some grass fed butter or fresh fruit and enjoy.

Bacon and Egg Salad

Servings: 4

Ingredients

- 6 hard-boiled eggs

- 4 pieces of bacon

- 2 medium onions, chopped

- 2 tbsp. Low Fat Mayonnaise

Directions

Place a medium sized skillet on a medium flame and add the olive oil to it. When the oil gets a little warmer, you will need to add the bacon to the skillet and let it turn brown and crispy. While the bacon is warming up in the skillet, cut the eggs into smaller pieces and add them to a medium sized mixing bowl and add the cooked bacon to it next. Mix these ingredients well together and add the onions to the bowl and continue to mix it well. Add the mayonnaise to the bowl and ensure that the mayonnaise holds the ingredients in the bowl well together to ensure that the salad is well made. Store this bowl in the refrigerator and eat it cold the following morning.

Banana Bread

Ingredients

- 1 teaspoon vanilla

- 4 bananas

- Pinch of sea salt

- ½ cup coconut flour

- 1 teaspoon baking powder

- 4 eggs

- 1 teaspoon baking soda

- 1 tablespoon cinnamon

- 4 tablespoons of melted grass-fed butter

- ½ cup almond butter

Directions

1. Preheat oven to 350 degrees F. Combine eggs, banana, grass-fed butter and nut butter in a blender and blend until smooth then add in cinnamon, coconut flour, baking powder, baking soda, sea salt and vanilla then mix well.

2. Pour the batter into a silicon pan that has been greased well. Bake in the preheated oven for around an hour or until a toothpick inserted in the center comes out clean. Remove from oven onto a cooling rack and let it cool then you can slice.

Pumpkin Pancakes

Servings: 2

Ingredients

- 1 egg

- ½ tsp. dried basil

- ½ tsp. dried parsley

- Salt and Pepper to taste

- ½ pumpkin, shredded

- ½ cup almond flour

- 1 tbsp. Butter

Directions

Take a small mixing bowl and add the shredded pumpkin to it along with the almond flour and the basil. Add the parsley, salt and pepper to the bowl and mix the ingredients well together. Add the egg to the bowl and mix the ingredients well together. Make a few patties with the dough you have. Take a medium sized pan and add the butter to the pan. Once the butter has melted, add the patties to the pan and cook them well on both sides. Once they have turned brown, serve them hot!

Coconut and plantain pancakes

Servings: 1

Ingredients

- ¼ teaspoon of baking soda

- ½ very ripe plantain (peeled and sliced)

- ¼ cup of coconut water

- A pinch of Himalayan or refined salt

- 3 whole eggs

- ¼ cup of coconut flour

- ¼ teaspoon of chai spice

- ¼ teaspoon cream of tartar

- *Garnish ingredients*

- 1 tablespoon of refrigerated coconut milk

- 1 tablespoon of unpasteurized honey

- 1 tablespoon of organic and toasted coconut shavings

Directions

Preheat the oven to 350 degrees F. Add all the ingredients you have except the garnish ingredients into a food processor and blend until they mix well. Leave the batter for some minutes to let the coconut flour thicken nicely. As your batter is resting, place your skillet over medium high heat and add a little amount of coconut oil. When the oil heats up, add like ¼ cup of the batter on the skillet or something close to that, which will be enough for one of your pancakes. Cook as you observe the edges. When the top starts becoming a little dull and matte and the edges appear cooked, flip it over and cook it until the whole batter turns golden. When it's done, place it in the oven set on low temps to keep it warm as you cook the other pancakes. When you are through, you can garnish with the coconut and honey then enjoy!

Macadamia Waffles with Fruit Syrup

Servings: 6

Ingredients

For the waffles

- ¾ teaspoon baking soda

- ¼ teaspoon of salt

- ½ teaspoon vanilla extract

- ½ cup coconut milk

- 3 eggs

- 3 tablespoons of honey

- 3 tablespoons of melted coconut oil

- 3 tablespoons and 1 teaspoon of coconut flour

- 1 cup raw macadamia nuts

- *Ingredients for the fruit syrup*

- ½ teaspoon of lemon juice

- 2 pitted and sliced peaches

- ¼ cup of honey

- 2 pitted and sliced plums

- ½ teaspoon of vanilla extract

- ½ cup of pitted cherries (can be fresh or frozen)

Directions

Place a saucepan over medium heat and add in all the syrup ingredients. Simmer for about 15 minutes and make sure to keep the heat constant and low to drain out all the juices perfectly from the ingredients. Before the 15 minutes are through, start preparing the waffles. Heat a waffle iron in advance on the lowest setting. Starting with the liquids, add all the waffle ingredients in a blender and blend. Start by blending on low for about thirty seconds and then another 30 seconds on high. When it's perfectly combined and smooth, spoon some batter in the preheated waffle iron (should be half way full and spread all over the mold). Cook for a maximum of 1 minute on low and make sure there is no steam from the cooking machine and the waffles come easily out of the machine before removing them. Keep the cooked waffles in an oven for warmth before you are done. When the syrup is thickened, enjoy it with the waffles.

Banana Pancakes

Servings: 1

Ingredients

- 2 tablespoons of chunky almond butter

- 2 bananas

- Dark chocolate chips (optional)

- 4 eggs

Directions

1. Mash the bananas in a large mixing bowl then combine with almond butter and then blend this with eggs in the bowl. Mix this well and then scoop about a quarter cup of this mixture then transfer it to a hot flat pan or griddle over medium heat. When bubbles appear, flip and cook for another 1-2 minutes.

2. Top each pancake with a sprinkle of dark chocolate chips (the darker the better), if you desire, then serve and enjoy.

3. This won't need any toppings but you are free to top with fresh fruits for extra sweetness and prepare sugar-free bacon as a side dish.

Chapter 6: Paleo Lunch Recipes

Glazed Pork Tenderloin

Servings: 2

Ingredients

- 2 pounds Pork Tenderloin

- 3 tbsp. Maple Syrup

- 3 tbsp. olive oil

- 3 tbsp. Balsamic vinegar

- 3 tbsp. dried thyme

- 2 tsp. paprika

- Salt and Pepper to taste

Directions

Preheat the oven to 200 degrees Fahrenheit. You have to make the marinade for the pork. Make use of every ingredient in the list mentioned above except for the pork and mix them well to create the marinade. You will need to ensure that there are absolutely no lumps in the mixture that you have made by using a whisk. Place the pork on a large plate and cover it well with the marinade that you have made. Coat the sides of the pork well with the marinade. Leave the marinated pork in a plastic bag and leave it in the freezer for a few hours. Once you have let it marinade for seven hours, place the pork on a baking sheet which has been coated with parchment paper and leave the tray in the oven. Leave the pork to bake in the oven for an hour. Pour the remaining marinade into a saucepan and place the pan on a low flame. When the marinade has started to thicken, turn off the flame. If the pork has cooked well enough, you will need to add it to the thickened marinade and coat the pork well. Leave the pan in the oven for another few minutes and leave it aside to cool. Roast a few vegetables and serve it with the pork.

Kale Caesar Salad with Cherry Tomatoes

Servings: 4

Ingredients

- 4 whole eggs

- Punnet of cherry tomatoes, halved

- 1 large brown onion, peeled and sliced thinly

- 1 teaspoon coconut oil

- Juice of ½ lemons

- 10 rashers of bacon

- Large bunch of kale leaves

- 3 tablespoons nutritional yeast

For the dressing

- 4 tablespoons mayonnaise

- 6 anchovies, chopped finely

- 3 tablespoons olive oil

- 1 clove garlic, grated

- ½ teaspoon Dijon mustard

Directions

1. Boil water in a small saucepan then heat the coconut oil in a frying pan and then add in bacon rashers and cook each side for a few minutes or until crispy. Remove to a chopping board then add in the sliced onion into a pan and cook this for few minutes or until it is softened and lightly golden. Proceed to add in 4 eggs to boiling water then cook this until slightly firmer than soft boiled eggs or for about 6 minutes. Proceed to rinse the eggs under cold water then peel.

2. While onion, bacon and eggs are cooking, prepare the kale. Tear the leaves away from the stalks and slice very thinly. Add to a large bowl and drizzle with lemon juice to soften the kale.

3. To prepare the dressing, mix all the ingredient in a small bowl then slice some bacon rashes into small pieces then add kale and the salad dressing and then toss through with the use of tongs or just by hand. Do this until well combined and to ensure that your kale is coated evenly.

4. Add cherry tomatoes, cooked onions and nutritional yeast (or grated Parmesan) and toss through gently. Serve in bowls topped with halved egg and an extra anchovy or two.

Poblano Peppers Stuffed with Guacamole

Servings: 4

Ingredients

- ¼ teaspoon salt

- 1 cup thinly sliced hearts of romaine

- ¼ cup chopped fresh cilantro

- 2 ripe avocados (halved and pitted)

- 5 medium Poblano peppers

- 3 tablespoons red onion- finely chopped

Directions

Preheat your broiler on high. Place the Poblano peppers on a fitting baking sheet. Place them 3-4 inches away from the source of the heat, and allow them to broil. Cook for about ten minutes or until the outer skin of the peppers darkens and then becomes blistered and turn them only once or twice if necessary. Once they are cooked, place them in a large bowl with a towel covering them and allow them to cool. Peel all the peppers but leave the stems attached. To a medium bowl, spoon out all the avocados and mash them together coarsely. Add in some salt, cilantro, and onions and stir them for a moment until they are well combined. Chop one of the Poblano peppers into the avocado mixture, and stir. Slit the walls of the remaining peppers, and take out the seeds. Take your prepared guacamole, add it equally in the four Poblano peppers and enjoy.

Coconut Curry Butternut Squash Soup

Servings: 4

Ingredients

- 1 large shrimp

- 1 tablespoon coconut oil

- 1 medium butternut squash

- 2 cups chicken or vegetable stock

- 3 teaspoons red curry paste

- ½ tablespoon fresh ginger

- Paleo adobo seasoning (blend 1/8 teaspoon ground turmeric, ¼ teaspoon black pepper, ½ teaspoon oregano, ¼ teaspoon garlic powder, 1 ½ tablespoons coarse sea salt)

- Freshly chopped cilantro

- 1 (14 ounce) can coconut milk

- 2 tablespoons coconut oil

- 1 tablespoon arrowroot powder

- 2 teaspoons coconut crystals (or raw honey)

- 1½ teaspoons coarse sea salt

- 1 small yellow onion

- 1 garlic clove

Directions

1. Add coconut oil to a pot placed over medium high heat. Chop the onion, ginger, and garlic then add into the pot and cook as you stir occasionally for around 5 minutes or until the onions are translucent.

2. Mix the arrowroot powder, salt, coconut crystals, and the curry paste and add them in the onion mixture and stir. Allow them to cook for one more minute before adding the broth, squash and coconut milk and broth and turn the heat to high. Reduce the heat to low when it boils and then let it simmer for 20-25 minutes more.

3. As it simmers, peel and then devein the shrimp and finally dust it with adobo seasoning. Place a pan on medium heat and add coconut oil to the pan before adding the shrimp. Let it cook for 5-7 minutes while stirring. Remove the shrimp from the heat when it turns pinkish everywhere and opaque. Then blend the squash mixture until its smooth. Add both the shrimp and cilantro (for garnish) on top of shrimp and serve immediately!

Poached Eggs with Curried Vegetables

Servings: 3

Ingredients

- 3 large eggs

- ½ tsp. white vinegar

- ½ tsp. red pepper (crushed)

- 1 cup water

- 8-ounces can chickpeas (drained)

- 2 medium zucchinis (diced)

- ½ pound button mushrooms (sliced)

- 1 tbsp. yellow curry powder

- 2 cloves garlic (minced)

- 1 large onion (chopped)

- 2 tsp. extra-virgin olive oil

Directions

Place a medium sized skillet on low flame and add the olive oil to the skillet. Once the oil has become hot, you will need to add the onions to the skillet and sauté them till they have turned golden brown and have become translucent. Now add the garlic to the skillet and cook it for thirty seconds. Add the curry powder and continue to mix the ingredients well together. Make sure that the powder has covered the onions and the garlic well. Add the mushrooms to the skillet and cook them well. Once the mushrooms have released all the liquid they have on the inside, you will find that they have become tender which will make them easier to cook. Add the water, the chickpeas and the crushed red pepper and bring all the ingredients to a boil. Once they have started to boil, add the zucchini to the skillet and let it cook. Start to reduce the heat and cover the ingredients while you let the ingredients cook well together. When the zucchini has become tender, you will need to move the skillet off the heat and let the ingredients cool. Take another saucepan and add the water, up to three inches deep, and bring it to a boil. Reduce the heat and crack the eggs and add the vinegar. Make sure that you let the ingredients cook for a minimum of ten minutes before you remove the eggs from the pan. Add the eggs to the skillet and cook the eggs along with the vegetables for ten minutes. Serve it hot!

Beef and mixed vegetable Stir Fry

Servings: 2

Ingredients

- ½ lb. beef

- 1 tbsp. coconut oil

- ½ cup onion minced

- 1 cup broccoli chopped

- ½ tbsp. sesame seeds

- 1 tbsp. green onion chopped

- ½ cup chestnuts sliced

Directions

You have to start cleaning the beef and then cut it into pieces which are equal in size. Take a pan and place it over a low flame and add the coconut oil to the pan. When the oil has heated, you will need to add the beef to the pan and cook it till the beef has turned brown in color on every side. Set the pan aside and let the beef cool. Take another pan and add the remaining oil to the pan. Add the onions and the broccoli to the pan and let them both cook till the onion has turned light brown and is translucent. Once the broccoli has started to wilt, you will need to add the mixture to the pan containing the beef and cook them together for a few minutes. You could add numerous vegetables to the pan if you choose to. Serve it hot.

Chicken curry salad

Servings: 4

Ingredients

- 1 heaping tablespoon curry powder

- 2 cups green grapes

- ½ cup almonds (silvered)

- Sea salt to taste

- 4 chicken breasts

- 2 tablespoons of honey (or more)

- 1/3 cup Paleo mayo

- Black pepper (to taste)

Directions

Use a piece of aluminum foil to line your baking sheet. Arrange your rack where the chicken will be set 2 inches from the source of the heat, then set the broiler on high. Rinse the chicken and remove any excess fat on it. Place the chicken side by side in the baking sheet and add sea salt and black pepper to taste. Place the baking sheets with the chicken in the oven. Allow it to bake for 14 minutes and remove it to cool when it's done. Then cut the chicken into small squares using a knife and mix the pieces with the grapes and the slivered almonds using a spoon in a mixing bowl. In another bowl, mix the Paleo mayo, curry powder, and honey until the mixture combines perfectly. Mix the mixture into the bowl containing the almond mixture grapes and chicken and enjoy.

Vegetables Roasted in an Oven

Servings: 4

Ingredients

- 3 tablespoons olive oil

- ½ teaspoon pepper

- 1 zucchini (cut into 1 inch pieces)

- 1 yellow summer squash (cut into 1 inch pieces)

- 1 teaspoon salt

- 1 red onion

- 1 red and yellow bell pepper (cut into 1 inch chunks)

- 1 pound of asparagus- cut into 1 inch pieces

Directions

Preheat the oven to 450 degrees F. Meanwhile, put a roasting pan over heat and add some oil. Add in all the vegetables and add then the salt and pepper to taste. Spread the vegetables all over the pan in one single layer. Let them roast for 30 minutes or until they are tender and brown as you check on them and stir occasionally. Let it cool for a while and serve while warm!

Chapter 7:
Paleo Dinner Recipes

Herbed Salsa and Grilled Chicken
Servings: 4

Ingredients

For the chicken:

- 1 teaspoon garlic, minced

- 2 boneless and skinless chicken breasts (8 ounces each)

- 2½ tablespoons extra virgin olive oil

- 2 ½ teaspoons chili powder

For the salsa:

- ½ teaspoon sea salt

- 1/3 cup of chopped fresh chives

- ¼ teaspoon of freshly ground pepper

- ¼ teaspoon of hot sauce (or to taste)

- ¾ cup of corn kernels (fresh or frozen)

- ¾ cup of chopped bell pepper (red or green)

- 1½ cups chopped tomatoes

- 1½ tablespoons of red wine vinegar (or more)

- 2 teaspoons of fresh chopped oregano

- 1/3 cup chopped of fresh parsley or cilantro

Directions

Add the cilantro or parsley, oregano, pepper, hot sauce, chives, vinegar, and salt in a food processor and combine with a cup of tomatoes. You have to process the mixture until its pureed and then add the bell pepper. Pulse it five times and transfer it to a non-reactive bowl like a glass bowl. Add the ½ cup of tomatoes remaining and corn and stir them together. Then cut the chicken diagonally into four equal parts. Combine in a bowl ½ cup of the salsa, 2 tablespoons of liquid drained from the salsa, garlic, chili powder, and 1 ½ tablespoons of oil. Add the chicken in the mixture and roll it inside until it's perfectly coated, cover it and put in a refrigerator. Heat the grill to a medium high heat then pat dry the marinade off the chicken with paper towels. Grease the chicken with oil and place them on a wire rack. Grill for about 10-15 minutes and turn the chicken once. Once done, serve with reserved salsa and enjoy.

Paleo Spaghetti

Servings: 8

Ingredients

- 1 large onion, chopped and diced

- 3 cloves garlic, minced

- 1 pound ground grass-fed beef

- ¼ cup chopped bacon

- Optional heavy cream (makes the sauce less acidic)

- Optional salt and pepper to taste

- 2 teaspoons dried oregano

- 2 tablespoons tomato paste

- 1 bay leaf

- 3 carrots, diced

- The equivalent of 2 cans whole meaty tomatoes

- Fresh parsley for garnishing

- 2 large Spaghetti squash

- 2 tablespoons olive oil

- 2 celery sticks, diced

Directions

1. Heat a large Dutch oven or pot and add olive oil. Cook the ground beef and bacon for about 5 minutes. Remove the meat with a slotted spoon and set aside.

2. Use the same oven or pot to cook carrots, celery, garlic, onion and oregano. Cook the vegetables until soft. Add the tomatoes, ground beef, tomato paste, bacon and bay leaf. You can break the tomatoes a bit, but the cooking process will break them anyway. It's optional to season with salt and pepper. You can also add some chili or hot pepper flakes for more heat. Bring to a boil and then reduce to a simmer for about 45 minutes.

3. Meanwhile, preheat the oven to 350 degrees F. Cut your spaghetti squashes in half lengthwise then remove and discard the seeds. Put the halves cut side down on a baking sheet and put in the oven for about 28 to 35 minutes. Check them for doneness with a fork at around 25 minutes. Make sure not to overcook them because they will become mushy and won't make pastas. Once the Bolognese sauce is well cooked, proceed to add about ½ - 1 cup heavy cream to make your sauce less acidic.

4. Pour a generous amount of the sauce directly on the squash halves so that they form their own bowl or you can scrape the inside out with a fork to form spaghetti-like pastas and serve on a plate with the sauce. You can add some grated pastured and grass-fed cheese on top and broil in the oven for about 5 minutes if you desire.

5. Garnish with fresh parsley and enjoy!

Taco Pie

Servings: 4

Ingredients

For the pie crust

- ¼ cup melted butter (or clarified butter)

- 1 teaspoon salt

- 1½ cups almond flour

For the pie filling

- 1 chopped avocado

- 1 pound of ground beef (grass fed)

- 1 red bell pepper (sliced)

- 1 tablespoon of olive oil

- Sea salt and a pinch of freshly cracked black pepper (both to taste)

- 1 cup of chopped lettuce

- ½ onion-chopped

- ½ cup of homemade barbeque sauce

Directions

Start with the pie crust. In a large bowl, combine the almond flour, butter, and salt. Blend the mixture until the dough forms. Switch the dough to a 9-inch pie plate and flatten it. Preheat your oven to 350 degrees F. Place a skillet on medium high heat and add the oil. Add onions and sauté them until they are translucent. Add the beef to the onions and fry until the beef cooks perfectly. Add barbeque sauce to the beef, season it with salt and pepper to taste. Let the beef cook for two more minutes and take the skillet off the heat when through. Place the cooked beef on top of the piecrust and put it in the oven for about 30-35 minutes. Take your taco pie out of the oven and garnish it with chopped lettuce, bell peppers, and slices of avocado and enjoy!

Smoky Mexican Tortilla-Less Soup

Servings: 4

Ingredients

- 7 ounces tomato paste

- ½ teaspoon chipotle powder

- ½ teaspoon sea salt

- 8 ounces of cooked and shredded chicken

- 2 teaspoons cumin

- 1 finely diced red bell pepper

- 1 small onion finely diced

- 32 ounces of homemade broth (beef or chicken)

- 1 roasted and diced Poblano pepper

- 2 tablespoons of coconut oil (or substitute with bacon fat)

- 2 teaspoons coriander

- ¼ teaspoon of black pepper (to taste)

- 2 stalks of celery- finely diced

- ½ cup finely diced carrots

Ingredients for garnish

- Avocado slices

- ¼ cup chopped cilantro

Directions

Put a large soup pot over heat and add the coconut oil to melt. Add the onions and let them cook until they are brown then add, the roasted Poblano peppers, celery, carrots, and diced bell pepper. Add the black pepper and salt to taste, chipotle powder, coriander, and cumin. Stir until it is combining and then leave it to cook for a few minutes. Add tomato paste and the broth and stir then heat the mixture slowly for about 20 minutes for the flavors to combine. Add the chicken in the mixture to heat it through. Add garnish of your choice and enjoy!

Pork chops with mushrooms

Servings: 4

Ingredients

- 8 ounces of white button mushrooms

- ½ cup of chicken broth or stock

- ½ teaspoon of dried rosemary

- 8 ounces of baby Bella mushrooms (cremini)

- 1 sliced onion

- 1 tablespoon of olive oil

- 4 bone in center cut pork chops

- 3 cloves of garlic (minced)

- Salt and pepper to taste

Directions

Add oil to a pan over medium high heat and add the pork chops after seasoning them with pepper and salt. Allow them to cook for 3 minutes on each side. When it's cooked put it aside. Add the onions and garlic after reducing the heat to medium. Cook until they are soft and add the mushroom and rosemary. Cook for 7 minutes and then add the broth and let it cook until it simmers. Slightly reduce the heat and then add the pork and cook for 8 minutes. Add salt and pepper (to taste) and then add the pork to the mushroom mixture and serve.

Chapter 8:
Paleo Dessert Recipes

Quick and Easy Dark Chocolate Pudding

Servings: 4

Ingredients

- 10 oz. can low or full fat coconut milk

- 2 cups unsweetened cocoa powder (dark)

- 1 cup maple syrup

- 2 tsp. vanilla extract

Directions

In a large mixing bowl, add the milk and the cocoa powder and mix them well together. Make sure that there are absolutely no lumps in the mixture when you whisk it. Now, add the maple syrup to the bowl to sweeten the mixture. Again, whisk the ingredients well to ensure that there are no lumps at all. You will need to taste the mixture in order to ensure that the balance is maintained. Transfer this mixture to a skillet and place it on a low flame. When the skillet is on the flame, you will need to stir it continuously while it is boiling and thickening. Remove the skillet from the heat and add the essence to the mixture. Mix it well and leave the pudding to cool. Transfer the pudding into an air tight container and store it in the refrigerator. Serve it cold with a scoop of vanilla.

Instant Strawberry Ice Cream

Servings: 4-6

Ingredients

- 1 pound unsweetened frozen strawberries

- 14 ounces of coconut milk

- ¼ teaspoon liquid stevia extract

- ½ tablespoon lemon juice

Directions

Place all the ingredients in your food processor. Run it until all the strawberries are well grinded. Refrigerate for a few minutes the serve and enjoy.

Fig and Cherry Bites

Servings: 18 mini cherry bites

Ingredients

- 10 dried Kalamata figs

- 3 cups dried cherries

- 2 cups of mixed nuts (preferably hazelnuts, walnuts and almonds)

- 2 cups dark chocolate chips

- 1 tsp. Cinnamon

- 2 tsp. Vanilla extract

- 2 tbsp. Maple syrup

- 2 cups unsweetened shreds of coconut

Directions

Take a baking tray or a cookie sheet and line it well with parchment paper. Make sure that the sides have been greased well with butter or with coconut oil. In a large mixing bowl, add the shreds of coconut and leave that bowl aside. If you find that the shreds are not very fine, process them or blend them and leave them aside. Ensure that each shred of the coconut is of the same width. Blend the cherries and the nuts together in the food processor or a regular blender. It is best if you chop the nuts into halves or smaller pieces before you put them in the blender or the processor. Add the maple syrup and the dried figs to the food processor and ensure that a sticky paste is made from processing all the ingredients together. Add the cinnamon and the vanilla extract to the paste in order to enhance the flavor. If the paste is too sticky for your liking, you will need to add a little water to the paste in order to reduce the stickiness. Make sure that you are able to spread the mixture out well. If you find that you are unable to do so, you will need to process the ingredients once more. Now add the chocolate chips and the shreds of the coconut to the mixture. Make this spread into smaller scoops and dip them in the chocolate chips and the coconut shreds. Ensure that they are covered all over with the coconut shreds. When they have been coated well, transfer the balls into the cookie sheet and let them bake at 180 degrees Fahrenheit for ten minutes.

Apple Spice Cookies

Yield 9 large cookies

Ingredients

- ½ apple diced

- 1 cup unsweetened almonds butter

- 1 teaspoon cinnamon

- 1 egg

- ¼ teaspoon ground cloves

- 1 teaspoon fresh ginger, grated

- 1/8 teaspoon nutmeg

- 1 teaspoon baking powder

- ½ teaspoon salt

- ½ cup raw honey

Directions

1. Preheat the oven to 350 degrees F. Combine almond butter, baking soda, egg, salt and honey in a bowl and mix until nicely incorporate then add apple ginger, spices and stir to combine.

2. Scoop a spoonful of the batter into a baking sheet and ensure you leave an inch or two between the cookies because they will spread.

3. Bake in the preheated oven for ten minutes then remove the cookies from the oven and allow them to cool for around ten minutes. Continue to cool the cookies on a cooling rack.

Beet Banana Brownies

Servings: 4

Ingredients

- 2 bananas

- 2 red beets, cooked

- 2 tablespoons honey

- 1 small 75% dark chocolate bar

- 1 teaspoon baking powder

- 1/3 cup almond flour

- ½ cup unsweetened cacao powder

- ½ cup chocolate protein powder

- 2 eggs

Directions

Mix all the ingredients in food processor except the dark chocolate and process until smooth. Stir in the dark chocolate bits then pour this into a pan that has been well greased then bake at 325 degrees F for around 40 minutes.

Blueberry Cream Pie

Servings: 8-10

Ingredients

Crust:

- 1 teaspoon almond extract
- 1 tablespoon lemon zest
- 2 tablespoons coconut oil
- ½ cup honey
- ½ teaspoon cinnamon
- 3 cups almonds
- Pinch of sea salt

Filling:

- 1 can coconut milk, chilled
- 1/3 cup honey
- 1/3 cup freshly squeezed lemon juice
- 2 teaspoons kosher plant-based gelatin that has been dissolved in two tablespoons hot water
- 4 blueberries for serving

Directions

1. Place the cinnamon and almonds in a food processor then process until you get the texture you want. Add the other crust ingredients and pulse until you have a sticky dough. Now pat the crust into a pie plate.

2. For the filling, mix the gelatin and water then add lemon juice. If the gelatin is clumpy, place the mixture in hot water to melt again. Pour coconut milk in an electric mixer then add honey and mix until peaks form. Add gelatin mixture to whipped cream then fold in. Pour the filling into the crust. Chill for around 4 hours until set then serve with the blueberries.

Banana Ice Cream

Servings: 10

Ingredients

- 2 teaspoons vanilla extract

- ¼ teaspoon stevia

- 1 cup cream

- 2 cups half & half

Add ins:

- ½ cup chopped pecans

- ¼ cup crushed and drained pineapple

- 1 banana, sliced thinly

- ½ cup toasted coconut flakes

- ¼ cup chopped 80% cocoa chocolate par

- ½ cup pitted and sliced cherries

- 1 cup sliced strawberries

Directions

1. Mix the dairy sweetener and vanilla in a bowl then make your ice cream depending on your ice cream maker instructions. If your ice cream maker allows, you can add the fruits nuts and other extras towards the last few minutes.

2. Serve and top with coconut flakes.

Chapter 9:
Paleo Slow Cooker Recipes

Slow Cooker Sweet Potatoes Mash
Servings: 4

Ingredients

- ½ teaspoon of allspice

- 1 tablespoon of ground cinnamon

- 1 teaspoon of ground nutmeg

- 1 cup of pure apple juice

- 2 pounds of sweet potatoes (peel and cut them into ½ inch slices)

- ¼ teaspoon ground cloves

Optional ingredients for garnish:

- Honey

- Pecans

Directions

Place the sweet potatoes in a slow cooker together with ½ cup of apple juice and desired spices. Leave them to cook on low for 4-5 hours. When the potatoes are cooked well, use the hand blender to mash them while in the slow cooker. Add the remaining ½ cup of apple juice and season with the nutmeg and cinnamon. Garnish with honey or pecans and enjoy.

Slow cooker roast chicken & gravy

Servings: 8

Ingredients

- Kosher salt

- Freshly ground pepper

- ¼ cup of white wine (or ¼cup of extra chicken stock)

- 1 teaspoon of tomato paste (or to taste)

- 4-5 pounds of organic kosher chicken

- ¼ cup chicken stock

- 6 cloves peeled garlic

- 2 medium onions-chopped

- 2 tablespoons of ghee

- Any of your preferred seasoning

Directions

Chop all your vegetables and melt the ghee in a skillet over medium heat. Sauté the onion and garlic and then add the tomato paste. Cook for about 10 minutes or until they are slightly translucent and then add both the pepper and salt to taste. Deglaze the pan using chicken stock or white wine and then transfer everything in the pan to a slow cooker. You can then dry off the chicken and season it with salt, seasoning and pepper. Add it in the slow cooker (breast side down) and let it cook on low for 4-6 hours. When the chicken is cooked, let it rest for twenty minute as it cools. De fat the braising sauce and blend with any seasoning in an immersion blender to come up with the gravy. Rip the chicken with your hands and serve with gravy.

Chunky Chicken Vegetable Stew

Servings: 6

Ingredients

- 1 large onion

- 1 yellow bell pepper

- 1 sweet potato

- ¼ bundle of kale

- 1 tomato

- 8 ounces of tasty mushrooms

- 1 pound of carrots

- 3-4 pounds of whole organic chicken

- 1 green bell pepper

- 1 winter squash

- 2 cups of chopped cabbage

Directions

Add the chicken to the middle of the slow cooker and chop the veggies around it. Season with your own desired seasonings and add around 2 cups of water. Cook for about 9 hours on low then fifteen minutes before eating, add the kale to prevent it from over cooking.

Slow Cooker Sausage Stuffed in Peppers

Servings: 4

Ingredients

- 2 teaspoons of dried oregano

- 1 small handful of fresh minced basil

- ½ head of garlic-minced

- 5 assorted bell peppers (green, red or yellow)

- ½ head of cauliflower-grated or chopped

- 2 teaspoons of dried thyme

- 1 small white onion (medium diced)

- 8 ounce can of tomato paste

- 1 pound of ground Italian hot sausage

Directions

Chop off the tops of the bell peppers and keep them aside and then seed the peppers. Add chopped cauliflower, basil, minced garlic, dried herbs and onions into a mixing bowl and mix the ingredients using your hand. Place a skillet on heat and when it's hot enough, add the sausage and let it cook until brown. Add the sausage and tomato paste to the bowl with the cauliflower and mix it again by hand. Fit the mixture into the bell peppers and place them in a slow cooker. Lightly place the tops back on. Cook the peppers on low for 6 hours and serve when you are ready.

Crockpot Veggies

Servings: 2

Ingredients

- 1 large sweet potato- peeled and chopped into cubes

- ½ cup of peeled garlic gloves

- 2 bell peppers cut into large chunks

- Oil (choose healthy oil)

- Salt

- 1 teaspoon of Italian seasoning-or any other seasoning of your choice

- 3 small zucchini (cut them into thick slices)

Directions

Add all the vegetables into the slow cooker after greasing it everywhere inside. Season the vegetables with some healthy oil, salt, and herbs. Stir until all the veggies are evenly seasoned. Cook the veggies on high for 3 hours stirring once in every hour. When they are cooked through, pour out the liquid but don't discard it (it's sweet also). Serve the veggies on 2 plates and enjoy.

Chapter 10:
Paleo Shakes and Smoothies

Banana berry molasses smoothie
Servings: 2

Ingredients

- 1 tablespoon molasses

- 4 ice cubes

- 1½ cups mixed berries, frozen or fresh

- ¾ cup of water

- 1 banana

- ½ cup coconut milk

Directions

Place all the ingredients in a blender. Run the blender until all the ingredients combine perfectly. You could add water to attain your desired consistency. Pour into a glass and enjoy.

Chocolate-Cinnamon Cherry Smoothie
Servings: 2

Ingredients

- 4 ice cubes

- 1½ cups of fresh or frozen cherries

- ½ cup of coconut milk

- 2 tablespoons of unsweetened cocoa powder

- 1 banana

- ¾ cup of water

- 2 teaspoons of cinnamon

Ingredients

Toss all ingredients into a blender and puree until smooth and creamy. You could also add water if you prefer a thin smoothie. Divide the smoothie into 2 cups and drink up.

Pineapple and Citrus Smoothie

Servings: 2

Ingredients

- ½ teaspoon nutmeg

- 1 teaspoon turmeric

- 1½ cups frozen or fresh pineapple chunks

- 1 orange- peeled and quartered

- ½ cup coconut milk

- 1 banana

- ¾ cup water

- Juice of 1 lime

- 4 ice cubes

- 1 tablespoon ginger

Directions

Add all the ingredients into a blender and blend until creamy and smooth. Serve and drink up.

Pumpkin Pie Smoothie

Servings: 2

Ingredients

- 1 ½ frozen bananas

- 1 ½ cups almond milk (unsweetened)

- ½ teaspoon of vanilla extract

- 1/8 teaspoon of nutmeg

- 1/8 teaspoon of cinnamon and another 1/8 for garnish

- ½ cup of pumpkin puree

- 1 teaspoon of maple syrup

- 1/8 teaspoon of ginger

- 1/8 teaspoon of all spice

Directions

Add all the ingredients except the 1/8 cinnamon reserved for garnish to the blender and then blend on high until creamy and smooth. Pour the smoothie into a large glass, garnish with the cinnamon, and enjoy.

Acai Boost Smoothie

Servings: 2

Ingredients

- 1 ½ cups of frozen blue berries

- 1 ½ cups of organic acai juice

- 1 frozen banana

- ½ cup of coconut meat (fresh)

Directions

Add all ingredients to a blender and then run until smooth and enjoy.

Sunflower Chocolate Smoothie

Servings: 2

Ingredients

- 1 teaspoon of cacao powder

- 4 pitted Medjool dates

- 2 frozen bananas

- 1½ cups of unsweetened almond milk

- 2 tablespoons of organic sunflower seed butter-unsweetened

Directions

Add all the ingredients in a blender and set it on high. Blend until smooth and serve.

Green Fruit Smoothie

Servings: 2

Ingredients

- 1 frozen banana

- 1 cup of spinach

- 1 teaspoon of coconut oil

- 1 teaspoon of flaxseed

- ½ cup of frozen and seedless green grapes

- 1 cored green apple

- 1 ½ cups of coconut water

- 2 tablespoons of raw honey

Directions

Add all ingredients to a blender and blend until smooth.

Chapter 11:
Paleo Snack Recipes

Sweet Potato Tater Tots and Tomato Ketchup

Servings: 2

Ingredients

- 2 sweet potatoes

- ½ onions (diced)

- 2 tbsp. coconut flour

- 1 tsp. garlic powder

- 1 tsp. chili powder

- ½ tsp. salt

- ¼ tsp. ground pepper

- ½ cup coconut oil (for frying)

Directions

Take the potatoes and wash them and peel them well. Once they have been cleaned, cut them into small cubes. Take a skillet and add water to it. Place it on a medium flame and when the water boils, add the potatoes to the skillet and cook them till they are slightly soft. Remove the water and leave the potatoes to dry for a while. Now, add the onions and the potato cubes to a food processor and mince them. Transfer this mixture into a mixing bowl and add the garlic powder, the coconut flour, chili powder, salt and pepper. Mix the ingredients well. Remove the mixture and try to shape them into small cylinders or cubes using your hands. Leave the cylinders outside to dry. While they are drying, take a skillet and add the coconut oil to it. When the oil has warmed, separate the cylinders and fry them. Once they have turned golden brown, you will need to remove them from the skillet and place them on paper towels to soak out the extra oil. Serve them with tomato ketchup!

Lettuce Chicken Wraps

Servings: 2

Ingredients

- 2 Lettuce leaves

- ½ pound ground chicken

- ½ an ounce of mushrooms, finely diced

- 2 cloves garlic, minced

- ½ tbsp. sesame oil

- ½ tbsp. vinegar

- Salt and pepper to taste

Directions

Take a pan and place it on a low flame. Add the sesame oil to the pan. When the oil has heated well enough, add the ground chicken to the pan and cook the chicken well. When the chicken has cooked, add the mushroom to the pan. Let the mushroom become golden brown before you add the vinegar and the ginger to the pan. Mix the ingredients well together and add the salt and pepper to the mixture. Take a lettuce lead and fill it with the mixture you have just made and wrap it up. Serve it!

Homemade Blackberry Paleo Fruit Roll ups

Servings: 8 roll ups

Ingredients

- 1 ½ cups blackberry

- 6 – 7 leaves of mint

- ½ cup honey

- 1 tsp. lime juice

Directions

First, preheat the oven to 200 degrees Fahrenheit. Take a baking sheet and line it with blotting or parchment paper. Make sure that you grease the sides well with coconut oil. Take all the ingredients mentioned and process them either in a blender or a food processor. Ensure that the paste is extremely smooth and that there are absolutely no lumps in the paste that has been prepared. Pour the mixture into a tray and spread it all out evenly. Leave the tray in the oven for two hours and remove the tray only when you are certain that the mixture is dry and slightly sticky. Leave the tray to cool for thirty minutes and cut the spread into thick strips and begin to roll each strip. Store these strips in an air tight container.

Tangy Taco Salad

Servings: 2

Ingredients

- 2 cups shredded lettuce

- 1 cup onion diced

- 3 tbsp. black olives

- 3 green onions chopped

- 4 ounces ground beef

- 1 tsp. garlic powder

- 1 tsp. oregano

- 2 tacos

- Salt and pepper to taste

- 1 tsp. olive oil

Directions

Place a saucepan on a medium flame and add the olive oil to the pan. Once the oil has warmed, you will need to add the beef to the pan and start cooking it. Turn the flame a little lower and continue to cook the beef. When the beef has cooked well, you will need to add the seasoning to the pan and continue to mix the ingredients well together. When the ingredients have blended well together, add them to a bowl and toss them well together. Take the two tacos and fill them with the beef mixture you have made and add some more seasoning if you want. Serve it hot.

Cucumber Pancakes

Servings: 2

Ingredients

- ½ cucumber, shredded

- ½ cup almond flour

- 1 egg

- ½ tsp. dried basil

- ½ tsp. dried parsley

- Salt and Pepper to taste

- 1 tbsp. Butter

Directions

Take a small mixing bowl and add the shredded cucumber to it along with the almond flour and the basil. Add the parsley, salt and pepper to the bowl and mix the ingredients well together. Add the egg to the bowl and mix the ingredients well together. Make a few patties with the dough you have. Take a medium sized pan and add the butter to the pan. Once the butter has melted, add the patties to the pan and cook them well on both sides. Once they have turned brown, serve them hot!

Paleo Trail Mix

Servings: 1

This snack is something you would love to consume when you have come back from work or when you are at work! You would have been really tired after working for four or five hours straight and this meal would help you regain all the energy that you may have lost. It will keep you active and the advantage is that you would never have to cook! This is a mean meal!

Ingredients

- 3 cups whole almonds

- 3 cup whole cashews

- 1 cup raw pumpkin seeds

- 1 cup raw sunflower seeds

- 1 cup raisins, golden and dried

- 1 cup dried currants

- 1 cup dried blueberries

Method

Take a small mixing bowl and add all the ingredients to the bowl and mix them well together. You would not need any dressing and can add any other ingredient you would want to.

Seasoned Sea Weed

Servings: 2

Ingredients

- 3 tablespoons melted coconut oil
- 8 nori sheets
- Sea salt to taste
- Sesame oil to taste

Directions

Preheat the oven to 350 degrees and rub 1/8 of the oil on a nori sheet. Add sesame oil and sea salt to taste and do this for all nori sheets. Stack 2 equal piles of nori sheets, set them on a baking sheet and place them in the oven. Bake to about 4 minutes then break the nori to small pieces and serve.

Macadamia Nut Humus

Yields 1 ¾ cups

Ingredients

- 1 clove of garlic
- 1½ cups of macadamia nuts- coarsely chopped
- ½ teaspoon of sea salt
- 2 tablespoons of olive oil
- 2 tablespoons of lemon juice

Directions

Add all ingredients except salt in a high-powered blender and process. Add about ½ cup of water and sea salt and run the blender until smooth. Refrigerate for 30 minutes and serve with carrots or zucchini or any vegetable for a healthy snack.

Paleo Spicy Pecans

Servings: 8

Ingredients

- 2 egg whites

- 5 cups pecan halves

- ¼ cup raw honey

- ¾ teaspoon ground nutmeg

- 4 teaspoons cinnamon

- 1½ teaspoons ground ginger

- ½ teaspoon ground cayenne pepper

- ½ teaspoon ground cloves

Directions

Grease 2 baking sheets as your oven preheats to 250 degrees. Add the cloves, cinnamon, ginger, cayenne, and nutmeg in a bowl and combine. In a large bowl, whisk the egg whites until they are frothy. Add honey to the bowl and keep on whisking until perfectly combined. Add one cup of the nuts to the mixture with egg whites and then to the mixture of spices. Place the nuts on the sheets and then into the oven and let them bake until they are crisp rotating once. Repeat with the remaining four cups and enjoy!

Natural Fruit Roll Ups

Servings: 8

Ingredients

- 2 cups water

- 1 teaspoon cinnamon

- 4 cups of your favorite fresh fruits- pitted, cored and pealed then chopped

- 2 teaspoons lemon juice

Directions

Add fruits into a sauce pan and simmer for 12 minutes. Mash and add lemon juice and cinnamon then stir. Allow it to simmer for 10 more minutes until thick. Put mixture in a blender and blend until smooth. Line baking sheets with parchment paper and add mixture on top (spread out). Heat oven to 140 degrees and place the mixture to dry. Roll up your preparation in parchment paper and serve.

Sweet and sour meatballs with sauce

Yields 3 dozen

Ingredients

- 2 large eggs

- 1 tablespoon sesame oil

- 2 teaspoons of sea salt

- 2 small Vidalia sweet onions

- 1 ½ teaspoons of ground ginger

- 2 pounds of ground beef, pork or chicken

- ¼ cup of almond meal (with skins) or 2 tablespoons of coconut flour

For the sauce:

- 1/3 cup honey

- 3 cups tomato puree

- ¾ cup unsweetened pineapple juice

- ½ teaspoon onion powder

- 2 tablespoons apple cider vinegar

- ¼ cup tomato paste

- 1/3 cup coconut aminos

- 1 ½ teaspoons sea salt

- 2 tablespoons Dijon mustard

- ½ teaspoon ground ginger

Directions

Preheat your oven to 350 degrees and start by preparing the sauce. In a wide pot, combine all the ingredients meant for the sauce. Set it at low heat setting for a few minutes then at low medium until it simmers for about 45 minutes until the syrup thickens (it should simmer while uncovered). As you let it simmer, prepare the meat balls. Add the onions to a food processor and let them mince finely. Add the almond meals, oil, sea salt, beef, eggs and ginger and pulse it until it is perfectly combined. Use your hands to pinch some and roll it to a bite sized meatball. Prepare 2 rimmed baking sheets and set evenly your rolled meat balls. Let them bake for about 12 minutes and remember to turn them once as they cook. Once you are through, place the sauce and meatballs in a slow cooker and set it on low. Cover them until they are cooked through and enjoy!

Chapter 12:
7-Day Paleo Diet Meal Plan

Day 1

Breakfast

Coconut and plantain pancakes

1 cup blueberries

Lunch

Chicken curry salad:

4 chicken breasts

1/3 cup Paleo mayo

Black pepper to taste

2 cups green grapes

Dinner

Stuffed bell peppers:

1 pound ground beef or turkey

2 bell peppers (any color)

1 onion, chopped

2 garlic cloves, chopped, or garlic powder

1 can diced tomatoes (or 1 fresh diced)

1 zucchini, chopped

2 raw eggs

Pre-made guacamole or avocado

Your preferred spices (you can use cilantro, pepper, salt, chili, cumin or garlic)

¾ cup Spring Vegetable Salad

Snacks

150ml 100% coconut water

1 handful of macadamia nuts

5 strawberries

Day 2

Breakfast

2 slices Paleo Banana bread

1 tablespoon almond butter

1 cup green tea

Lunch

Barbecue pepper and eggplant salad (with your favorite seasonings):

2 red peppers

2 green peppers

2 large eggplants

2 hard - boiled eggs

Dinner

Slow cooker sweet potatoes mash

Dessert

Blueberry cream pie

Snack

Spicy Pecans

Day 3

Breakfast

2 Banana pancakes

1 cup green tea (unsweetened)

Lunch

Pumpkin rocket-salad:

2-3 cups peeled pumpkin chunks/strips (Butternut or Kent)

2 small beef fillet steaks

Tahini dressing

Rocket salad

Dinner

Chicken Curry Salad

Snacks

Handful of almonds

Carrots with macadamia nuts hummus

Day 4

Breakfast

Banana pancakes

1 cup coconut milk

Lunch

Chicken Curry Salad

Dinner

Paleo spaghetti

Dessert

Instant Strawberry Ice cream

Snack

1 handful of macadamia nuts

5 strawberries

Day 5

Breakfast

Eggs baked in avocado

1 green apple

Lunch

Lemon & garlic scallops:

¾ cup butter (or Ghee)

2 tablespoons lemon juice

2 pounds large scallops

3 tablespoon garlic, minced

Salt and pepper to taste

Serve the scallops on a bed of steamed or roasted vegetables

Dinner

1 serving Paleo almond chicken fingers (serves 4):

1 pound boneless, skinless chicken breasts

1 cup almond meal

2 eggs, lightly beaten

1 tablespoon paprika & ½ teaspoon garlic powder

1 teaspoon cumin

1 teaspoon cayenne pepper& 1 teaspoon black pepper

Dessert

Acai Beet Smoothie

Snack

An apple

Day 6

Breakfast

1 bowl nuts & berries

1 cup coconut milk

Lunch

Citrusy Shaved Zucchini & Sardine Salad:

1 medium zucchini, washed and shaved into ribbons (discard the inner, seedy core)

½ lemon juice

½ teaspoon sea salt

2 tablespoons extra-virgin olive oil

2 tablespoons chopped green onion

1 medium roasted pepper, sliced (or as much as you like)

1-2 tablespoons pumpkin seeds

100g tinned sardines

Dinner

Pork chops and mushrooms

Snack

Sunflower Chocolate Smoothie

Day 7

Breakfast

Tomato and egg stir-fry

1 cup green juice (choose the vegetables)

Lunch

Pork chops and mushrooms

1 pear

Dinner

Citrus roast chicken (serves 6):

1 whole chicken (about 4 1/2 pounds)

3 lemons or limes (if using limes, use 4)

5 tablespoons coconut oil (or lard, tallow, butter)

3 tablespoons grated fresh ginger

2 oranges

Sweet potato fries

Dessert

Pears poached in red wine

Snack

1 slice of melon

Bonus Chapter!

This chapter covers another seven day meal plan you could use to test whether or not the Paleo diet works for you! The advantage here is that you have two plans you could use to your benefit when it comes to planning your diet. This is the simplest plan and will be easy for you to follow when you are starting out on your Paleo diet. The plan given above can be used if you are able to stick through seven days! You can use the different recipes that have been mentioned in the book to your benefit and make your plans using these recipes since they are utterly delicious!

Day 1:

Breakfast – Zucchini Pancakes

Lunch – Glazed Pork Tenderloin

Snack – Lettuce Chicken Wraps

Dinner – Taco Pie

Day 2:

Breakfast – Banana Bread

Lunch – Beef and Mix Vegetables Stir Fry

Snack – Paleo Spicy Pecans

Dinner – Paleo Spaghetti

Day 3:

Breakfast – Banana Pancakes

Lunch – Coconut Curry Butternut Squash Soup

Snack – Natural Fruit Roll Ups

Dinner – Smoky Mexican Tortilla – Less Soup

Day 4:

Breakfast – Paleo French toast

Lunch – Chicken Curry Salad

Snack – Paleo Trail Mix

Dinner – Slow Cooker Sweet Potato Mash

Day 5:

Breakfast – Kale and Red Pepper Frittatas

Lunch – Poached Eggs with curried vegetables

Snack – Cucumber Pancakes

Dinner – Crockpot veggies

Day 6:

Breakfast – Scrambled Eggs

Lunch – Kale Caesar Salad with Cherry Tomatoes

Snack – Acai Boost Smoothie

Dinner – Chunky Chicken Vegetable Stew

Day 7:

Breakfast – Pumpkin Pancakes

Lunch – Vegetables Roasted in an Oven

Snack – Chocolate-Cinnamon Cherry Smoothie

Dinner – Slow Cooker Roast Chicken and gravy

Conclusion

Thank you again for choosing this book!

You would have learnt well about how the paleo diet helps you with becoming healthier and happier! I hope the paleo diet recipes plus the two 7 day paleo diet plan will be helpful even as you start your paleo diet journey. You could use these two plans as your blueprint before you start making your own plans. You have been given numerous recipes which are mouth – watering and will leave you wanting more.

The next step is to start preparing the meals as this is the only way that you can tell what you love and what you may not. Don't be afraid to try different combinations of food, as this is what will help you know what you prefer eating.

Finally, if you enjoyed this book, would you be kind enough to leave a review for this book on Amazon?

Click here to leave a review for this book on Amazon!

Thank you and good luck!

www.ingramcontent.com/pod-product-compliance
Lightning Source LLC
Chambersburg PA
CBHW062047280526
45788CB00003B/1136